Aerobic Yoga

THE COSMIC FOUNTAIN OF YOUTH WORKOUT

Aerobic Yoga

THE COSMIC FOUNTAIN OF YOUTH WORKOUT

Szabolcs Atzel-Bethlen
and Yvette Mimieux

JOURNEY EDITIONS
Boston • Tokyo

First published in 1997 by Journey Editions, an imprint of Tuttle Publishing, with editorial offices at 153 Milk Street, Boston, Massachusetts 02109.

Library of Congress Cataloging-in-Publication Data

Atzel-Bethlen, Szabolcs, 1944–
    Aerobic yoga: the cosmic fountain of youth workout / Szabolcs Atzel-Bethlen and Yvette Mimieux.
        p.   cm.
      ISBN 1-885203-40-3
      1. Yoga, Hatha.   I. Mimieux, Yvette.   II. Title.
  RA781.7.A85 1997
  613.7'046—dc21   97–4178
                                           CIP

Distributed by

USA
Charles E. Tuttle Co., Inc.
RR 1 Box 231-5
North Clarendon, VT 05759
Tel: (800) 526-2778
Fax: (800) FAX-TUTL

Southeast Asia
Berkeley Books Pte. Ltd.
5 Little Road #08-01
Singapore 536983
Tel: (65) 280-3320
Fax: (65) 280-6290

Japan
Tuttle Shokai Ltd.
1-21-13, Seki
Tama-ku, Kawasaki-shi 214
Japan
Tel: (044) 833-0225
Fax: (044) 822-0413

First Edition
05 04 03 02 01 00 99 98 97   1 3 5 7 9 10 8 6 4 2

Design by Cynthia Patterson
Printed in Singapore

Acknowledgements

I would like to express my thanks to all who have helped me write this book. Special thanks to Peter Ackroyd for giving me the chance and guidance; to my editors Isabelle Bleecker and Doug Oliver, whose dedication and direction greatly refined the manuscript. I am especially grateful to my art director, Cynthia Patterson, for her artistic vision and inspired style that brought poetry to this book. Many thanks to Raiko Hartman, the photographer whose untiring professionalism and remarkable technique created the beauty of the imagery. Also, to Mark Rosin and Barbara Greenleaf for their guidance. My special thanks to photographer Jim McHugh and journalist Nancy Nash for their help in presenting this book.

Words cannot express my appreciation to my co-author, Yvette Mimieux, for her inspiration, insights, and wisdom.

Contents

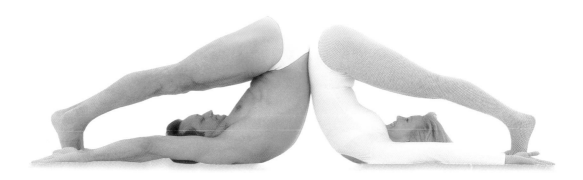

o n e

Introduction
A Yoga Workout for Today's World

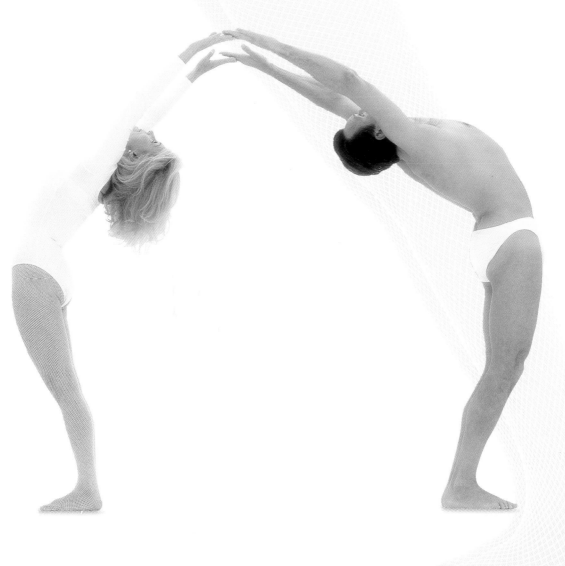

Why "Cosmic Fountain of Youth"?

For five thousand years people all over the globe have greeted the Sun, Moon, and Earth with symbolic rituals that acknowledge nature's awesome power. Beginning and ending the activity of the day, they set its rhythm as well. In ancient times these rituals offered a comforting stability in an often frightening world. Today similar rituals are an effective way to combat the stresses and anxieties of our modern era.

Over the centuries each culture has adapted a solar greeting to its own personality and pace of life. By adding the traditional yogic Salutation to the Sun to my own combinations of yogic poses, the Salutation to the Earth and Salutation to the Moon, I have created a yoga workout attuned to today's world. Because it acknowledges the Earth, Sun, and Moon, and promotes health, vigor, and long life, I call it the Cosmic Fountain of Youth.

How the Cosmic Fountain of Youth Workout Developed

When I was growing up in Eastern Europe, I was very much taken with martial arts. Although there were few outlets for my interest, I persevered and eventually became a martial arts expert, an initiate of the Kodokan Judo Institute of Tokyo. But as I continued to expand my sports repertoire to attain optimum fitness, I felt

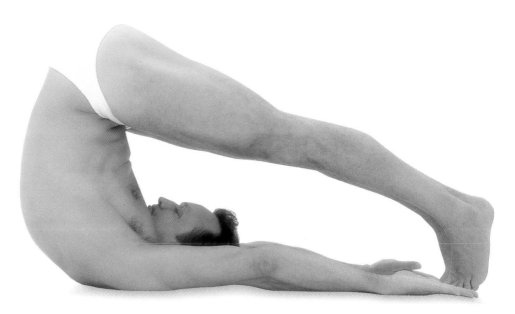

something was missing. That something, I discovered, was yoga.

As always when in the grip of a life-force idea, I went directly to the source, in this case India, home of this ancient practice. There I studied the sciences of stretching and breathing techniques (hatha yoga and *pranayama*) at yoga institutes in New Delhi and Calcutta and monasteries in the Himalayas.

Finally satisfied that I had mastered the ideal mind-body exercise, I returned to California to found the Yoga College of Beverly Hills, where I have taught for more than a decade. It was here that I developed my own unique fitness program that became the Cosmic Fountain of Youth.

Yin and Yang: The Dynamic Interaction of Opposites

assivity and activity, stillness and movement are universally recognized metaphors for the dualities that exist in the world and within ourselves. Externally, there are such opposites as female (yin) and male (yang), night and day, cold and hot. Internally, we speak of calmness and agitation, acceptance and rejection, and other dualities.

I believe there is a powerful energy in the dynamic interaction of opposites. That is what inspired me to create the Cosmic Fountain of Youth. By stretching and strengthening the muscles, relaxing and toning the body, and calming and stimulating the system, this workout harnesses the energy of these opposites.

What is new and different about the Cosmic Fountain of Youth is that in creating it I have synthesized the opposite essences of the two great cultures of India and China: the yin of hatha yoga and the yang of t'ai chi ch'uan.

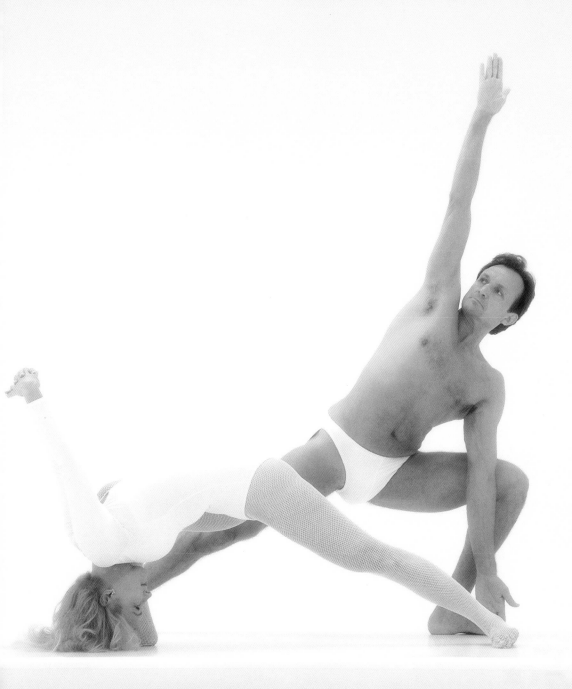

Hatha Yoga + T'ai Chi Ch'uan = Meditation in Motion

There are many forms of yoga and yoga systems. What most of us generally mean by "yoga" is properly called hatha yoga. Hatha yoga is the cornerstone of the Cosmic Fountain of Youth. It is a several-thousand-year-old mental-physical practice rooted in Indian culture. In simplest terms, hatha yoga is the practice of getting into certain positions and holding them in a statuelike manner. These "meditative" yogic poses give the body balance, flexibility, strength, and energy, and improve concentration, relaxation, and breathing.

T'ai chi ch'uan, or "supreme ultimate boxing," is the product of Chinese philosophy and culture. T'ai chi, as it is commonly called, is a system of continuous, fluid movements practiced to enhance health, fitness, and peace of mind. Although its origins lie in martial arts, the aspect of self-defense is secondary. In essence, t'ai chi is the path to attaining harmony with the universe and, thus, health, long life, and tranquility.

By combining the dynamic (yang) movement of t'ai chi with the static (yin) poses of hatha yoga I have added motion to meditation for a new aerobic yoga workout.

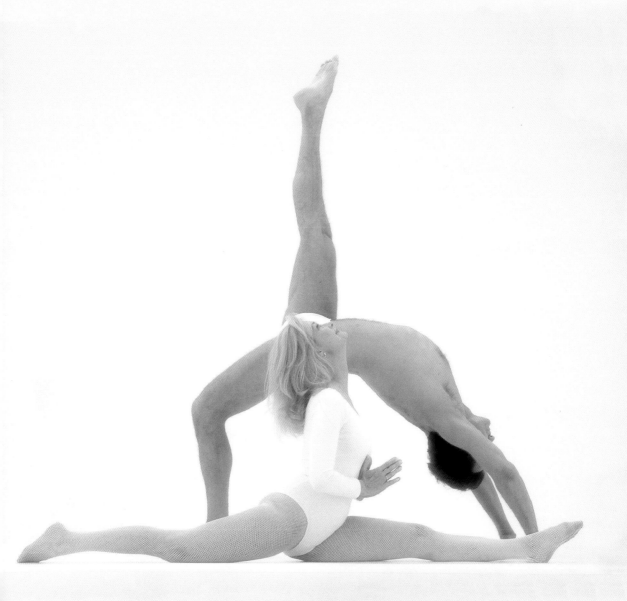

The Cosmic Fountain of Youth

The workout consists of three sets of exercises, the Salutation to the Earth, the Salutation to the Sun, and the Salutation to the Moon.

The Salutation to the Sun is an ancient exercise. For centuries it has been practiced at sunrise to release spinal tensions and stiffness accumulated during sleep. It is also an important cardiovascular and respiratory system stimulator. Though I reaped the benefits of this exercise for many years, over time I wished for a more challenging and varied cycle of poses.

Then, while in India, I came across a reference to the Salutation to the Moon. The poses of this exercise were not structured in any particular order, however, and they were quite similar to those of the Sun cycle. The greatest limitation of both cycles was that they were two-dimensional—neither had side stretches—and they were still predominantly for warm-up purposes. I realized that with my knowledge of yoga I could redesign the Salutation to the Moon to increase the variety and the intensity of the cycle.

To complement these cycles I created a totally new cycle with a lower degree of difficulty than the Sun and Moon cycles. I named it the Salutation to the Earth. Beginning with the moderate floor exercises of the Salutation to the Earth, continuing with the more difficult exercises of the Salutation to the Sun, and culminating in the intense exercises of the Salutation to the Moon, the three cycles together became my revolutionary exercise system, the Cosmic Fountain of Youth.

Who Will Benefit from This Book?

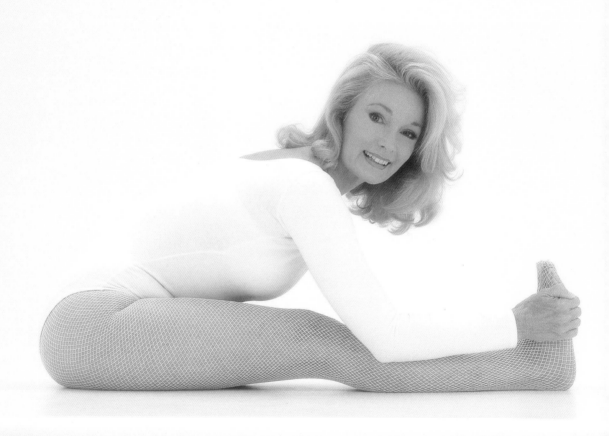

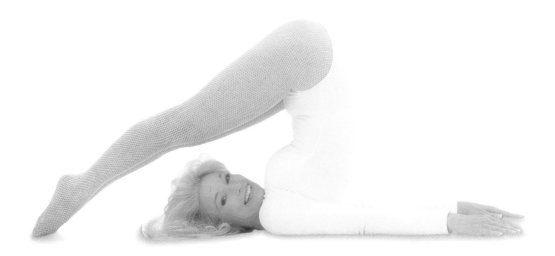

The Cosmic Fountain of Youth is designed for people of all ages and in all stages of physical proficiency. You can profit from the workout whether you are a yogi or yogini or have never taken a yoga class in your life. You will see progress whether you're in perfect health or you suffer from spinal, circulatory, or other health problems. And you will benefit whether you never exercise, just play sports on weekends, or are a professional athlete.

The secret to the all-encompassing benefits is the individual nature of the workout. *You* set the pace. *You* decide how often to practice. *You* plan the number of cycles. And *you* determine how vigorously you're going to do them.

How You Will Benefit

The Cosmic Fountain of Youth works all the major muscle groups, including those to which we rarely pay attention. A daily routine guarantees that you will realize the maximum benefit in the minimum amount of time. By vigorously performing the workout, you will achieve a superior level of aerobic fitness. You will be amazed at how quickly you experience improvement in your flexibility, strength, stamina, and controlled breathing.

In ten years of teaching I have seen these exercises bring dramatic results time and again. Because these exercises release stiffness and disperse energy blocks of the spine, neck, and back, my students have liberated themselves from aches, pains, fatigue, and even migraine headaches. As you go through the cycles you will revitalize, tone, and strengthen your body, mind, and spirit.

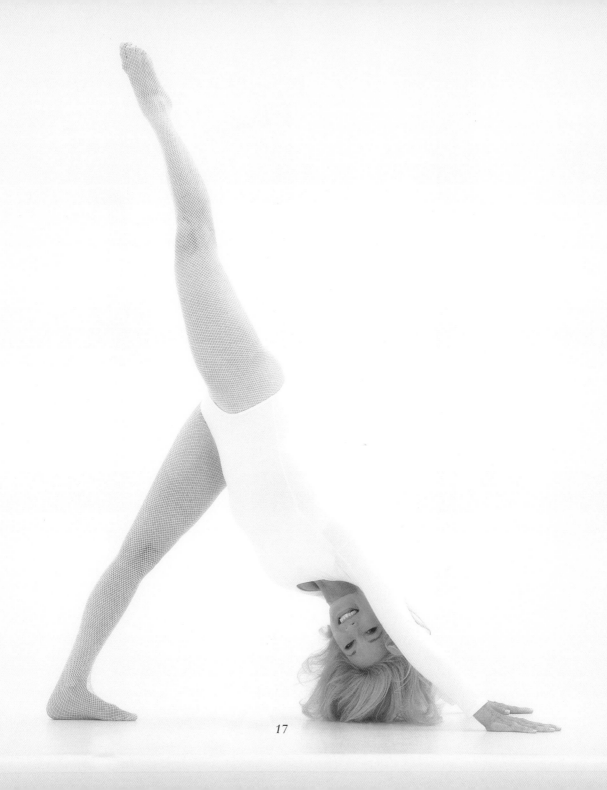

17

A Fountain of Youth

Aging is a complex biochemical, psychological, and physical process. As babies our bodies are free from tension, our skin is alive and free of wrinkles, and our breathing is perfect. We are vigorous and we regenerate quickly. In old age our bodies can become stiff and out of alignment, our range of motions can become limited, our skin dry and wrinkled, and our breathing short and shallow. Regeneration is slow and limited, and there is a lack of life force.

This deterioration, however, is not inevitable. Since the only factor of the aging process we cannot change is genetics, most of what we think of as the "normal" effects of aging can be prevented and controlled. Consistently practiced, the stretching and breathing exercises of the Cosmic Fountain of Youth can dramatically slow down, stabilize, and even reverse this deterioration.

How to Use This Book

Before you practice the cycles, learn the poses individually. When you start to put the sequences together, practice each pose slowly with the book in hand. In the beginning, you can interrupt the flow in order to collect yourself and execute the motions harmoniously. You can also rest between cycles if you are out of breath. You will find as you progress that you will be able to do the cycles easily and you will not have to—or want to—stop between cycles.

More Than Just an Exercise Program

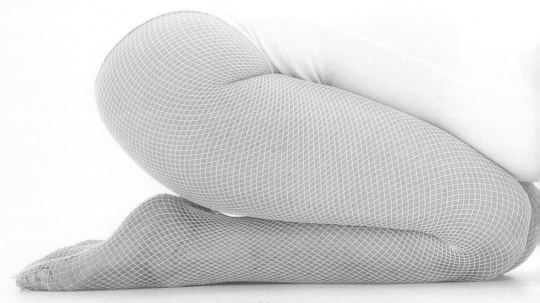

*A*s part of an ever-evolving personal exploration and self-improvement program, the workout has no specific end. It is a lifelong pursuit. The more you do it, the more centered, integrated, and balanced you will become physically, emotionally, and mentally.

Yes, you will gain firmer thighs and arms and a harder belly—but you will gain much, much more. You will be working on your body as an entity, not artificially isolating one muscle at a time. You will achieve a firm center, spirit, and core. Wholeness is what this workout is all about. Practicing the Cosmic Fountain of Youth Yoga Workout will put you on the path to a healthy, flexible body, sexual youth, and vigor.

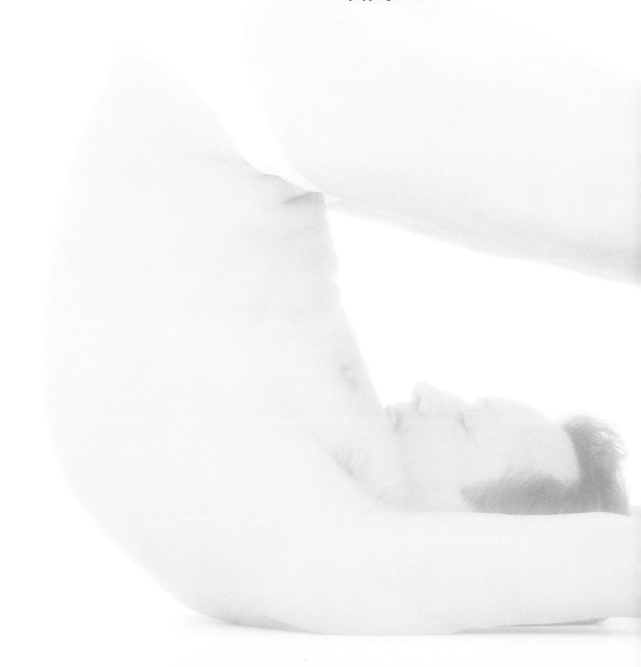

t w o

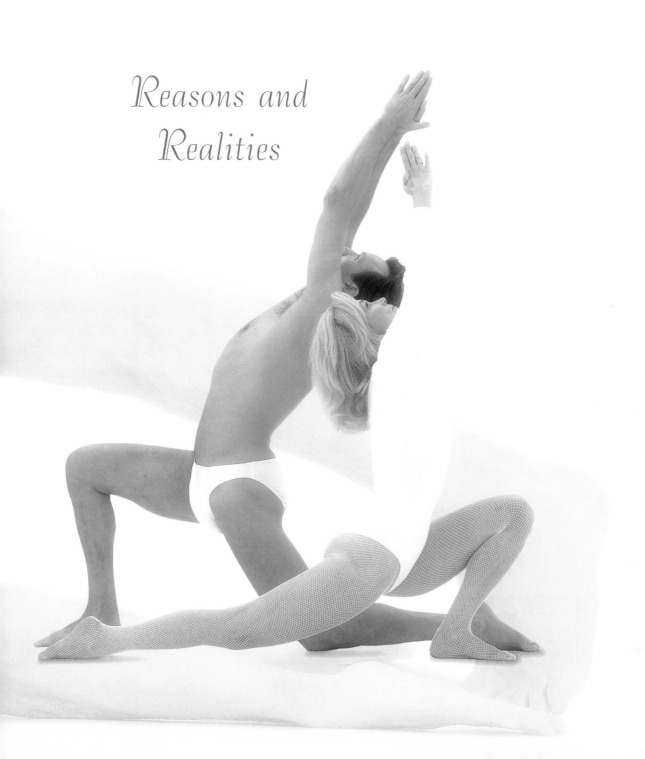

Reasons and
Realities

Breathing

$\mathcal{A}$ s you become more proficient in the Cosmic Fountain of Youth Yoga Workout, you will be able to concentrate on your breathing. Breathing is the most vital function of our existence. It is generally believed that breathing is automatic and beyond our control. But that is not true. We can actually change the rate and depth of our breathing pattern, increasing its efficiency and thereby our own energy. Breathing provides not only oxygen, but also *prana* or life force.

According to yogic tradition, prana is the energy permeating the universe at all levels. It is physical, mental, intellectual, spiritual, and sexual. It is cosmic energy. All energies are prana. It is the potential or latent energy in all beings. It is the primal cause of all activities. Prana is the breath of life.

In order to collect, conserve, and direct life force and oxygen efficiently, we have to improve our breathing. By properly practicing the workout, and with the help of yogic breathing exercises such as synchronized breathing, we can control inhalation and exhalation. Inhalation energizes the respiratory system. Exhalation disposes of the carbon dioxide, used lung tissue, and toxins. When proper, diaphragmatic breathing is achieved, life force or energy is distributed from the life center throughout the entire body.

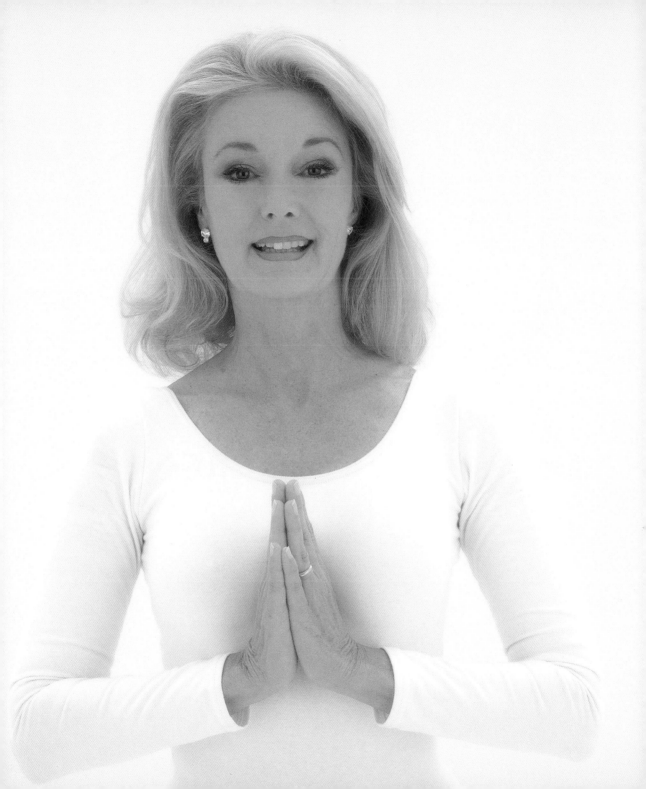

Yogic tradition teaches that the life center is located in the center of the body approximately two inches below the navel. We are born with a properly located life center and, as children, our breathing is controlled by the diaphragm, the flat, membranelike muscle that separates the chest from the abdominal cavity. But due to stresses and anxiety as we grow up, most of us develop a misplaced life center and lose the ability to breathe properly. By practicing the Cosmic Fountain of Youth we can alter our breathing pattern, increase our energy supply to its optimum, and bring the life center back to its proper location.

Correct breathing is always:

Even and deep. Short, uneven breaths lead to hyperventilation, which results in light-headedness, dizziness, and anxiety.

Continuous. Do not suspend your breath between exhalation and inhalation while doing the workout. Retention of the breath is applied only in yogic breathing exercises.

Effortless. There is no need to struggle with your breathing during activities. When you try too hard, you get tired quickly. Instead of forcing the timing of your inhalation and exhalation, let your breathing find its own rhythm, one that flows naturally.

Nearly soundless. The sound of breathing reflects its evenness, continuity, and effortlessness. Listen to your breathing during practice and relaxation.

Diaphragmatic. Using the abdominal muscles as you breathe allows your diaphragm to function correctly. During exhalation, your abdomen *must* contract. During inhalation, it *must* expand. You may check your breathing while standing or lying down by placing your palm on your abdomen with your thumb on your navel. As you breathe in, your palm should rise. As you breathe out, your palm should fall. Your goal is noticeable change without strenuous effort.

Through the nose. Breathe through your nose while practicing the Cosmic Fountain of Youth. If you feel tired, you might open your mouth during exhalation, but always breathe in through your nose. By inhaling through your mouth, the filtering, cooling, warming, moistening, and disinfecting functions of the nostrils are bypassed. Additionally, the inflow of air through your mouth will be uneven and shallow.

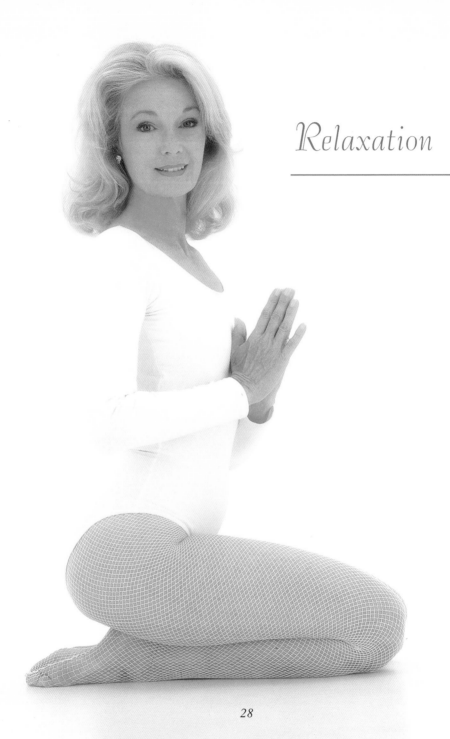

Relaxation

*P*hysical, emotional, and mental strains translate into muscular tension. Tension is detrimental to correct breathing. The Cosmic Fountain of Youth provides a method for releasing tension, thus enhancing correct breathing and harmonizing the functions of body and mind.

In order to relax, create the right conditions:

Abdominal breathing.

Correct poses. It is particularly important to maintain or restore the alignment of the spine. Any tension of the supporting muscles or deformation of the spinal column inhibits the natural flow of energy and correct breathing.

Calm mind. The mind must be free from distractions. It should be peaceful and serene.

Work toward two types of relaxation:

Physical. You can relax your muscles and internal organs by intentionally releasing tension. The Cosmic Fountain of Youth is an excellent way to accomplish this.

Mental. One of the easiest and most effective methods of achieving mental relaxation is to concentrate on your breathing. By directing your attention to breathing, you release and minimize tension.

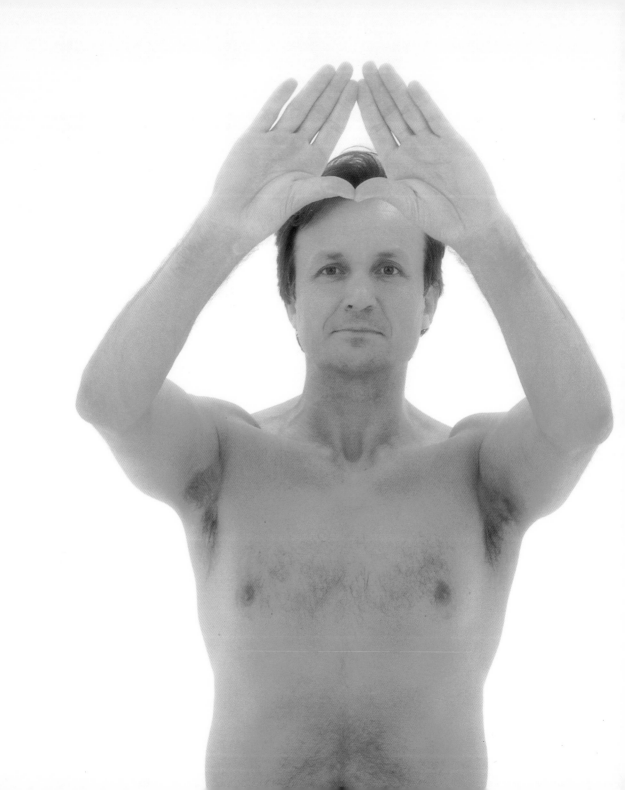

Concentration

Without any particular deliberation, all of us find ourselves focusing on one matter or another in the course of the day. But there is a higher level of concentration, one that brings us a greater sense of well-being, but obtaining it is an active pursuit. I refer to it as "conscious concentration."

In conscious concentration, the mind focuses on a single point. The simplest form of this activity is when the mind and eye are both aimed at a real object. At a more advanced level, concentration is held by images, prayers, or sacred sounds called *mantras*. The objects or reasons for concentration might vary, but they always result in increased mental clarity and willpower.

The Cosmic Fountain of Youth requires a simple form of concentration, during which the mind and vision are aimed firmly and persistently at a point of focus.★ When you are starting out, your point of focus will change often and arbitrarily, but with practice you will gradually consolidate it.

★*Since every pose has a specific point of focus, each time you change a pose, the point of focus will change as well.*

In this workout, concentration enhances the centering sensation. To maximize it, you should be aware of the distracting and debilitating nature of emotions and sound. Emotions awaken anxiety, and anxiety undermines the mental-physical balance you are trying to achieve. That is why your state of mind during the workout should be serene, but not rigid. Your goal is emotional neutrality; you want neither the high of elation and enthusiasm nor the low of anger and frustration.

Finally, you might find yourself holding your breath while concentrating. But I urge you to try to maintain an even, continuous, and deep breathing pattern. You will find it easier to ignore distractions if you focus on your breathing.

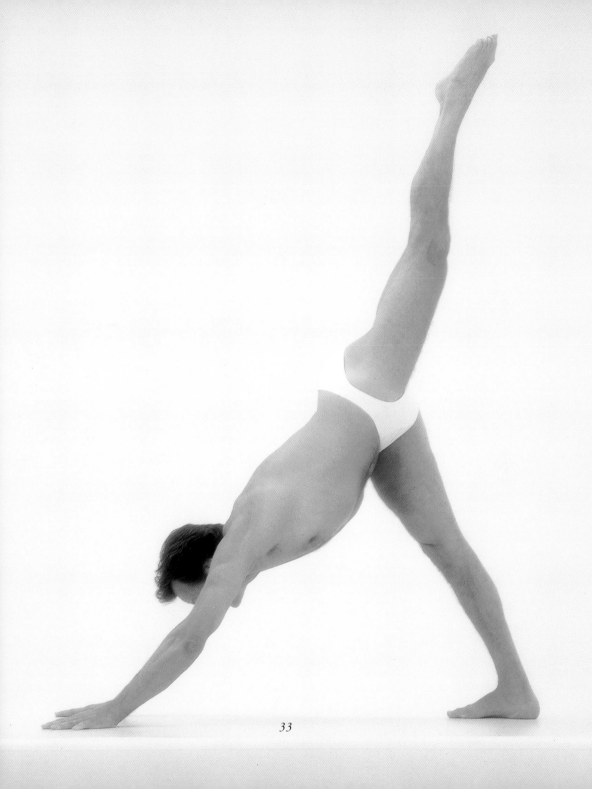

33

Balance

When you think of balance in connection with the Cosmic Fountain of Youth, you should think not so much of the ability to remain stable on one foot as about the goal of retaining equilibrium in your life. The essence of hatha yoga, on which the workout is based, is balance in every facet of life.

"Ha-tha" means Sun-Moon. It represents the duality of life, and it is also the embodiment of the balance and dynamic interaction of opposite forces. Yin-yang, relaxation-tension, flexibility-strength, passivity-activity, and static-dynamic are expressions of the same principle.

If you have ever engaged in sports you probably emphasized one aspect of your development over another, thereby creating a physical imbalance. Runners and joggers are usually stamina oriented and neglect to work on strength and flexibility. Bodybuilders work on their strength, but not on flexibility and stamina. And tennis players favor one side of the body over another.

By practicing the Cosmic Fountain of Youth, you will achieve balance between flexibility, strength, and stamina while developing both sides of your body equally.

You will begin the balancing process at the basic physical level. But with improvement of your physical balance will also come an improvement in your mental and emotional state. This principal law of psychosomatic unity has been well known in yoga for thousands of years. If you persist with the Cosmic Fountain of Youth routine, you will eventually reach a marvelous state of physical, emotional, and mental equilibrium.

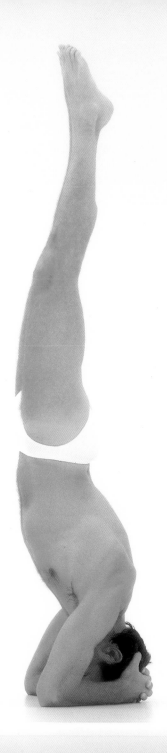

Execution of Technique

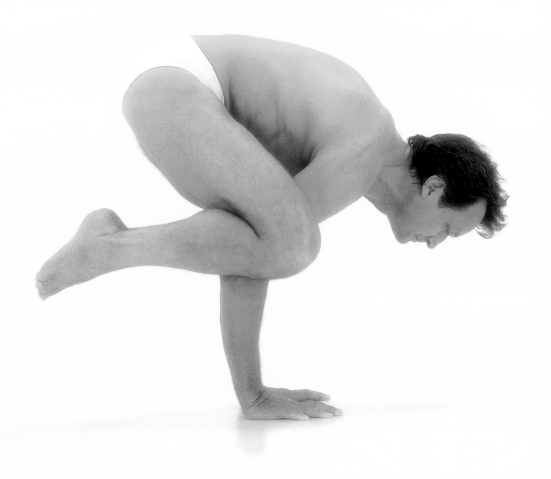

Your goal in the Cosmic Fountain of Youth Yoga Workout is a fluid, ever-unfolding series of movements.

The correct execution of the cycle is:

Even, continuous. When you start out, you might interrupt the continuity in order to collect yourself, regulate breathing, or regain balance and concentration. But remember to take up where you left off; it is not necessary to repeat the previous movement. In the same vein, if at first you have difficulty following the prescribed breathing pattern, by all means, breathe continuously. Just remember to follow the breathing pattern when entering or exiting a pose.

Controlled. If you lose concentration, balance, or strength as you go through the routine, take it in stride. Rather than berate yourself, simply double your efforts at concentration, and you will be back in control in short order. If you must stop in the middle of the routine, try to do so gracefully.

Synchronized. As time goes on you will be able to synchronize your motions with your breathing. In fact, the breathing will dictate and regulate the rhythm of your routine. If you practice in a group or with another person, synchronize your movements. This will further the atmosphere of harmony that is so much a part of the workout.

Graceful. Tension and rigidity will destroy the essence of all you are trying to achieve with the workout. Aim for ease and grace from the outset, understanding that these benefits will build with repeated practice.

Serene. Try to rid your mind of serious or troubling thoughts. You will maximize the benefits of the workout if you can maintain a natural, unforced calm.

Total. As you become more knowledgeable in your routine, you will see that the movements entering and exiting a position are important to the whole of the workout.

Try to perform the movements at a rate that is neither too slow nor too fast. Your guide should be the even, harmonious, "cosmic" speed of correct breathing. Sudden, jerky motions will interfere with the harmonious state you are trying to achieve, so do not rush through the routine. Initially, as you are learning, it is better to move at a rate you can control than to whiz through the exercises in fits and starts.

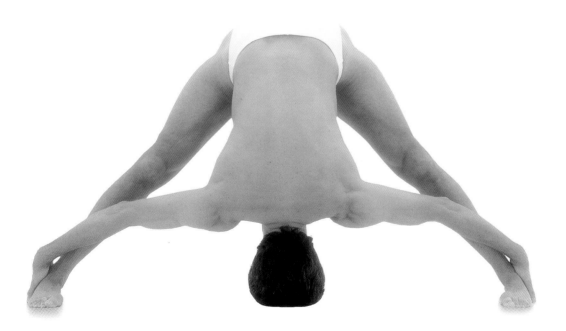

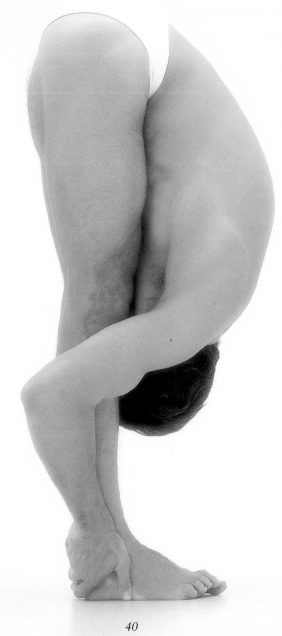

Stretching

Stretching is how we achieve flexibility, and it is one of the main elements of the Cosmic Fountain of Youth. Stretching is most beneficial when we combine physical pressure and mental relaxation.

The correct stretch is:

Moderate. If you find yourself shaking or vibrating excessively when you stretch, you are trying too hard. You are denying a sufficient blood supply to the muscles and building up tensions that obscure the feelings and sensations you are trying to get in touch with in this workout. Strong, excessive mechanical pressure not only causes excessive chemical reactions in the muscles, which results in stiffness and fatigue, but it also may invite injuries. If you feel pain while stretching, ease up or stop altogether. Heed this warning signal! Remember, moderation is the leading principle of the Cosmic Fountain of Youth.

Steady. Refrain from sudden, jerky motions.

Emotionless. Strive for a state of mind similar to that of an observer: free from personal involvement.

Controlled. Your breathing rhythm will determine the length of time it takes you to enter, hold, and exit the poses. Eventually, you will be able to do the exercises fluidly, without a break in motion.

Conscious. You can learn how to stretch the muscles not only by applying physical pressure, but by learning to relax the muscles voluntarily until they achieve better resting length.

Relaxed. The less anxious you are, the more effective your stretching will be.

Properly timed. Since the Cosmic Fountain of Youth is based on continuously flowing movement, you need not be concerned about holding the poses. The rhythm of your breathing will determine the duration of the stretch.

Total, complete. As you embark upon the exercises, do not isolate the muscles or parts of your body while stretching; instead engage the body in its totality. Every part of your body has to participate actively or passively; no part should be limp or out of alignment.

Frequency, Length, and Time of Practice

You may practice the Cosmic Fountain of Youth as often as you wish, because none of the movements places a strain on the body. To the contrary, they act as rejuvenators, a secret source of relaxation and strength whenever you feel like a pick-me-up.

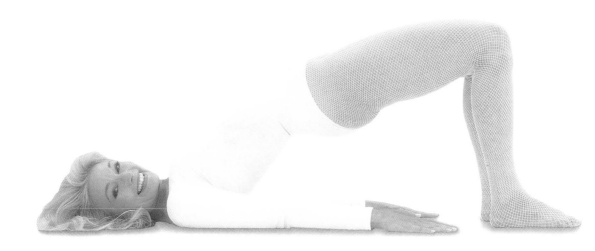

Daily Practice

Working out daily has many advantages, and I recommend that you make it a habit to get the maximum benefit from the routine. You will progress more quickly, you will remember the movements more easily, and the exercises will give structure to your daily routine.

Length of Practice

You may design the workout to fit your own schedule. On those days when you are pressed for time, you can accomplish the whole routine (and get something out of it!) in only eight minutes. That means completing two repetitions of each cycle moving at a moderate pace. Do this short routine if you oversleep or have only a few minutes to yourself between appointments. It is better to do less than to feel pressured—which would undermine all you are trying to accomplish with the workout. On other days, when you have more time, you can spend 12 minutes and do three Earth, Solar, Lunar repetitions, or 16 minutes and do four repetitions of each cycle. With each repetition, the stiffness will leave your body and you will feel looser, more relaxed, more alert, and more integrated.

Time of Practice

The time when you practice is entirely up to you, but I think that at least one of your daily workouts should be first thing in the morning. You are apt to be least distracted with the day's concerns when you wake up. The world is relatively quiet first thing in the morning, and you can concentrate on your movements and breathing without the clatter of daily activities.

Eating, Drinking, and Working Out

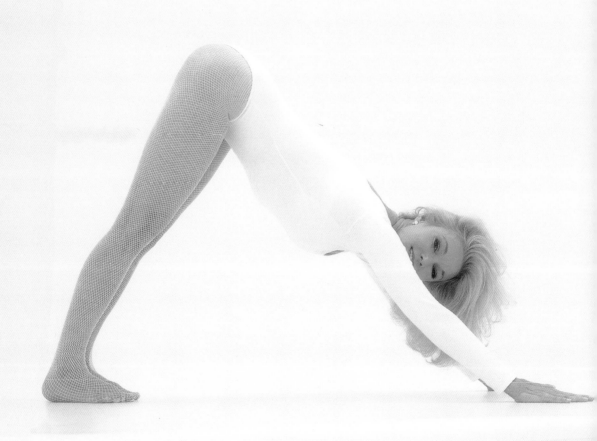

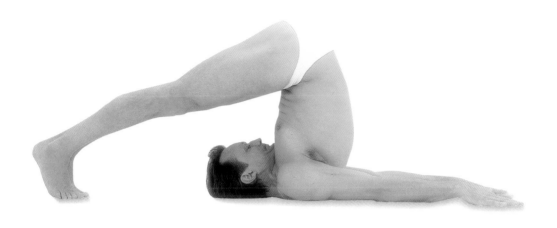

You have probably often heard that it is not a good idea to eat just before exercising. This precaution also pertains to the Cosmic Fountain of Youth. But did you ever wonder why? Here is the reason: When you put food and liquids into your digestive system, you are limiting the correct functioning of your diaphragm. Your breathing becomes shallow, and you exert undue pressure on your internal organs. On a full stomach, pressure from certain movements not only results in discomfort, but may also be harmful to internal organs. At the same time, the act of digestion takes blood away from your muscles and your brain, just when they need an increased supply of oxygen.

You should stop eating two to three hours before practice and stop drinking a half hour before working out. If your mouth and throat become dry as you go through the workout, take a small amount of water, but try not to make this a habit. And, of course, to get the most out of your workout, do not stop to eat!

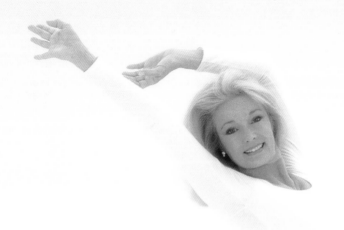
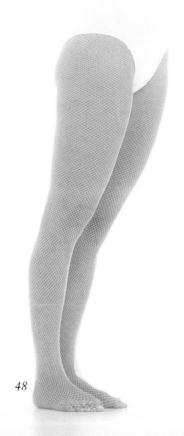

48

Injuries

As with all hatha yoga practice, the basic principles of the Cosmic Fountain of Youth are moderation and self-control. If you go only so far and so fast as your body allows, you will not injure yourself. In fact, unless you become impatient and start to push too hard, you have less chance of injuring yourself with this fitness routine than with almost any other.

What should you do if you should experience some unpleasant sensations during a prolonged workout? Common sense dictates that you ease up. Modify the movements that are making you uncomfortable, and chances are that you will work out the distress as you go along.

If the pain persists, of course, you'll have to call it quits for a while. Under no circumstances should you suppress pain artificially. If you can only continue to exercise by taking pain relievers or wearing bandages and braces, you will make the damage worse, and your injury will take longer to heal. Take a rest and allow nature to follow its course of repair and regeneration.

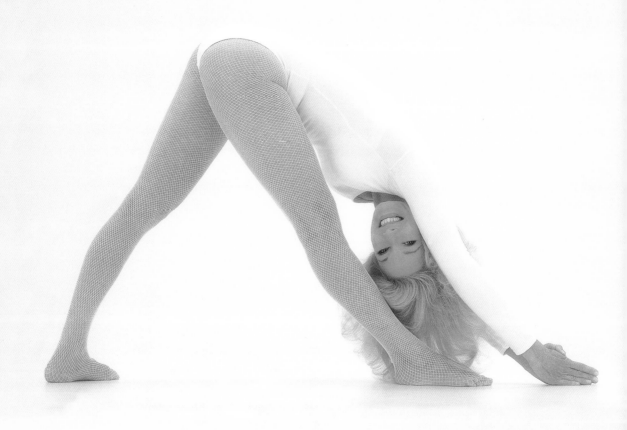

Practical Questions

Where should I set the thermostat?

It is best to practice the Cosmic Fountain of Youth at normal room temperature (65°), but if you are wearing light clothing, set the thermostat a bit higher to keep your muscles warm. You do not want them to stiffen up from cool air. If weather allows, practice in front of an open window or out of doors. I do not recommend that you do the workout in the hot sun.

What should I wear?

Wear a light and comfortable outfit for the workout, such as a leotard or a bathing suit. Take off your tight belt, because pressure on the abdomen will keep you from breathing correctly. And be sure to remove your watch and any jewelry.

Can I do the workout in a sauna?

Absolutely not! Avoid any place with exceptionally high temperature while working out. At first the heat might feel soothing, but soon it will sap your energy. Heat masks undue pressure and even pain, thus immobilizing the warning system that lets you know when you are overdoing it. It increases your heartbeat too, leading to exhaustion, hyperventilation, and dizziness. High temperature is also harmful to the respiratory system. If it is too dry, it damages the air passages, and if it is too moist, it fills the lungs, thus lessening your capacity for oxygen intake. It is absolutely untrue that if you practice in high temperature you will acquire greater stamina.

Should I be concerned about perspiring?

You will perspire to some extent while doing this workout. In moderation that is all to the good: perspiration has a cleansing and cooling function. But if you perspire excessively by forcing your movements, you will weaken rather than strengthen the cardiovascular system. The more you learn to relax during the workout, the less you will generate nervous perspiration.

Should I work out in front of a mirror?

Strict practitioners of yoga frown on performing the traditional poses in front of a mirror. I take a more relaxed view and see the mirror's value as a self-correction aid, especially when you are first learning the routine. As you advance, though, you should give up the mirror and rely instead on muscle memory to keep your body in proper alignment.

What is the ideal floor surface for the workout?

The best floor is more hard than soft, but avoid discomfort.

What should I do if I feel stiff?

In the beginning or when restarting a set after some time away from exercising, you may experience stiffness and unpleasant sensations, particularly on the second or third day. Do not give up! Rather, adhere to your routine, stretching gently until the soreness goes away. A hot bath or sauna after exercising also helps to loosen tight muscles.

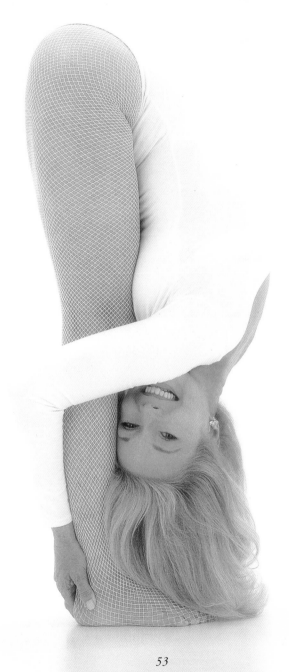

53

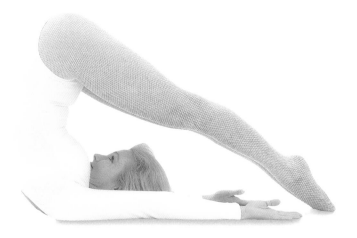

What does it mean if I have a headache or feel dizzy?

Hyperventilation, suspension or shortening of the breath, struggling, or sudden motions can bring on headache, light-headedness, or dizziness. These symptoms are natural for a beginner. The good news is that as you practice more, the movements will come more easily, your breathing will become more rhythmic, and these uncomfortable symptoms will disappear.

What if I experience muscle twitches, spasms, or cramps?

If you find that your muscles start to twitch, spasm, or cramp, you are working out too hard for too long a period of time. The discomfort you feel is a tension reaction. To relieve it, massage the tensed area. In the case of cramps, try some gentle stretching of the affected area. Since poses are not held in the Cosmic Fountain of Youth as they are in traditional hatha yoga, you should not experience the calf-muscle cramping that comes from prolonged pointing. But if you do, flex your toes and feet until the cramp diminishes. Then massage the tensed muscles. If you find you are experiencing spasms or cramps frequently, even without strong and long-held stretches, you might need to add more calcium to your diet.

What if I pull a muscle?

A "pulled" muscle is actually an injured muscle. If your distress is not too severe, massage the area that hurts. Try to continue your routine, but not to the point of provoking pain. If the muscle hurts a lot, place ice on it as soon as you can and stop stretching the muscle until it heals. Do not massage a severely pulled muscle.

Can anything be done for tendonitis?

If your ligaments and joints are tender or inflamed, avoid those movements that call them into play. You will probably heal quickly if you place ice on the affected area after practice. But if the inflammation persists, consult your physician about treatment.

How should I handle sciatica?

You can practice the Cosmic Fountain of Youth even with this condition if you avoid the poses that provoke it. If the pain does not diminish within two or three weeks, have your doctor check it out.

Suppose I suffer from back pain?

Then the Cosmic Fountain of Youth Yoga Workout is for you! Unless you have had back surgery or long-standing problems, you can perform the exercises at your own rate and see your flexibility improve. Gentle stretching is ideal for working out backaches, but if your problem is severe, please consult with your physician before embarking on this routine.

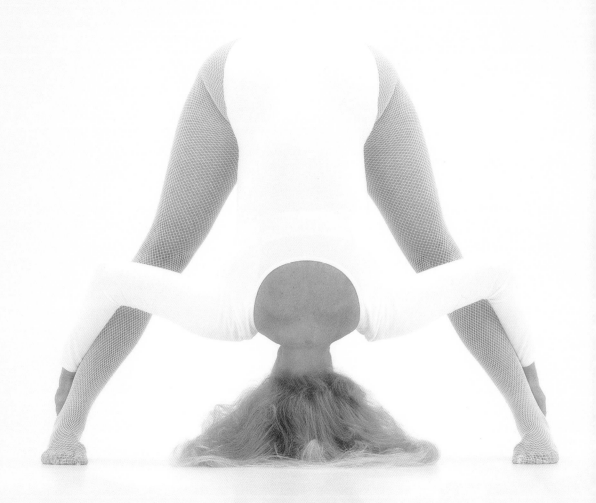

Can I work out while menstruating?

Yes, just decrease the intensity of your practice and avoid those poses in which your head and torso point toward the floor.

Will I be able to continue through my pregnancy?

Absolutely. In fact, it is advisable to engage in a stretching routine such as the Cosmic Fountain of Youth during pregnancy, but with decreasing vigorousness as your pregnancy advances. Experiment with modifying the poses and avoid working out on your stomach. As you gain weight, stretch moderately to avoid developing permanent stretch marks. If your back starts to ache, do some relaxing stretches to relieve the tension collecting there, as opposed to pushing through in a hard-driving routine. Of course, if you feel exceptionally fatigued, simply call it quits and rest for a while. After delivery, do not practice for two to four weeks, but you can and should go on with your controlled breathing even when physical exercise is not recommended.

What if I suffer from asthma or bronchitis?

You will be delighted by the improvement you see in these conditions as a result of committing yourself to this workout. Asthma and bronchitis are often improved dramatically by the regular and moderate practice of breathing exercises and hatha yoga.

Should I stop exercising if I have a cold?

That is not necessary. You can do the routine, but avoid group exercise and never, ever practice when you have a fever.

What if I cough while working out?

Sometimes you might experience a fit of coughing that cannot be explained by a cold or other obvious circumstances. When that happens don't be alarmed. It might be thought of as your body's spontaneous attempt to disperse tension from your chest and shoulders.

Why do I find myself yawning during practice?

As you well know, prolonged, frequent yawning is usually a sign of exhaustion. However, during practice or relaxation, occasional exaggerated involuntary breathing might occur. This may be a sign of deep relaxation, or it could be a signal that your breathing has become too shallow. In the latter case, the yawn acts as a substitute for deeper breaths.

Should I be concerned about fatigue?

If you feel totally depleted after this workout, you will have to modify the intensity of your routine. Ideally, the vigor of your motions should be perfectly matched with the strength of your body, leaving you feeling light and joyous at the conclusion of the exercise cycles.

A final word: Take all the little aches and pains of life in stride and see them disappear as you get deeper and deeper into your exercise routine. But if some troubling discomfort persists, no matter how mild, please have your doctor check it out.

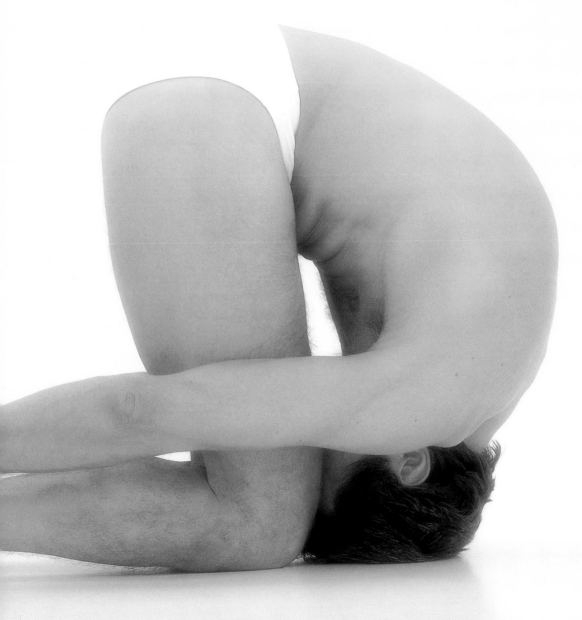

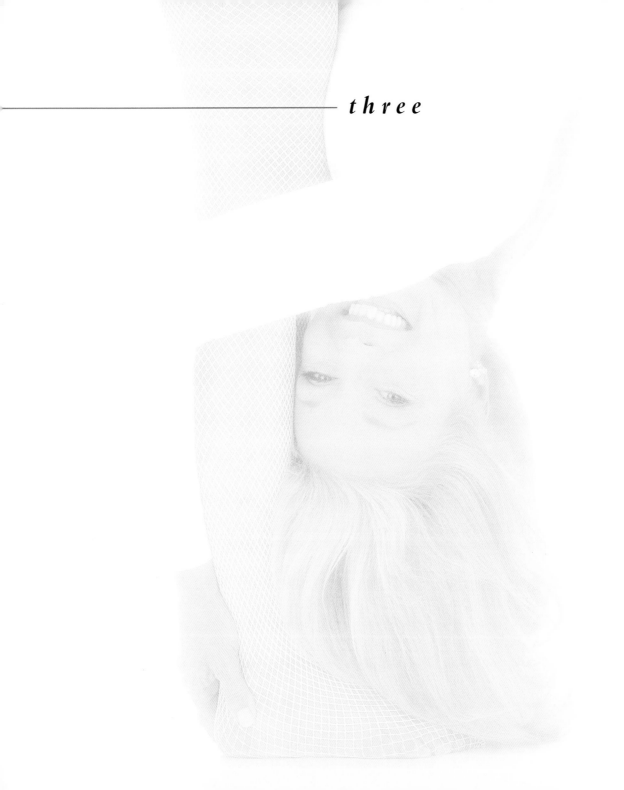

t h r e e

The Cosmic Fountain of Youth
Yoga Workout

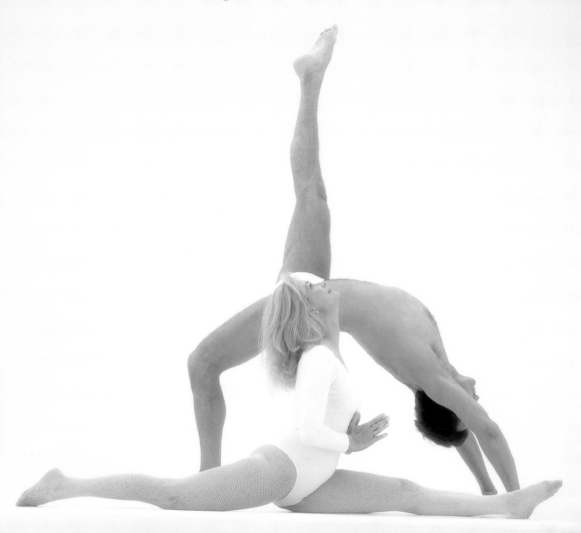

We always begin and end our practice with a breathing exercise that invigorates and prepares us for physical activity.

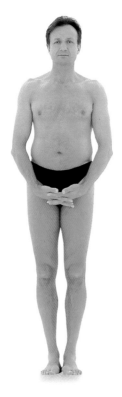

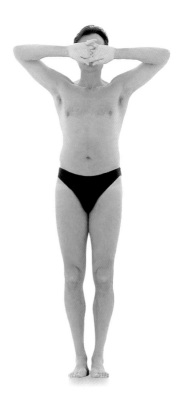

1. Stand with feet together, arms at your sides. Inhale-exhale as you bring your hands together and interlace your fingers, palms upward.

2. Inhale through your nose as you raise your arms, palms upward, close to your body. When your hands reach face level, rotate your palms outward.

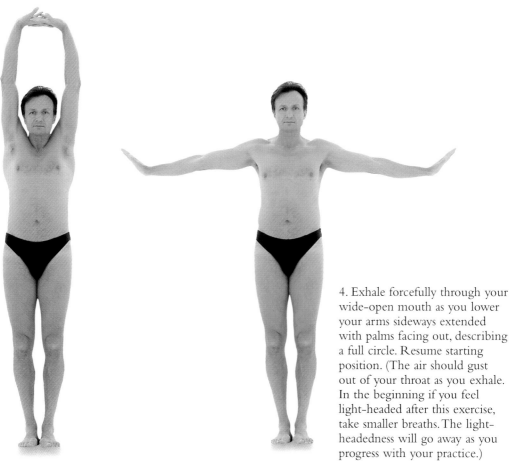

3. Continue to inhale, filling your lungs to capacity. Rotate your hands, stretching your straight arms, palms upward, over your head.

4. Exhale forcefully through your wide-open mouth as you lower your arms sideways extended with palms facing out, describing a full circle. Resume starting position. (The air should gust out of your throat as you exhale. In the beginning if you feel light-headed after this exercise, take smaller breaths. The light-headedness will go away as you progress with your practice.)

During inhalation your abdomen should expand; during exhalation it should contract.

Repeat the breathing exercise four to six times. Use the full capacity of your lungs to inhale and exhale.

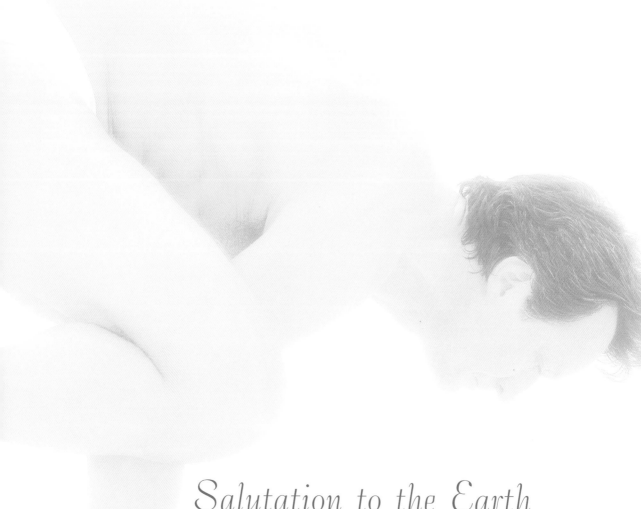

Salutation to the Earth

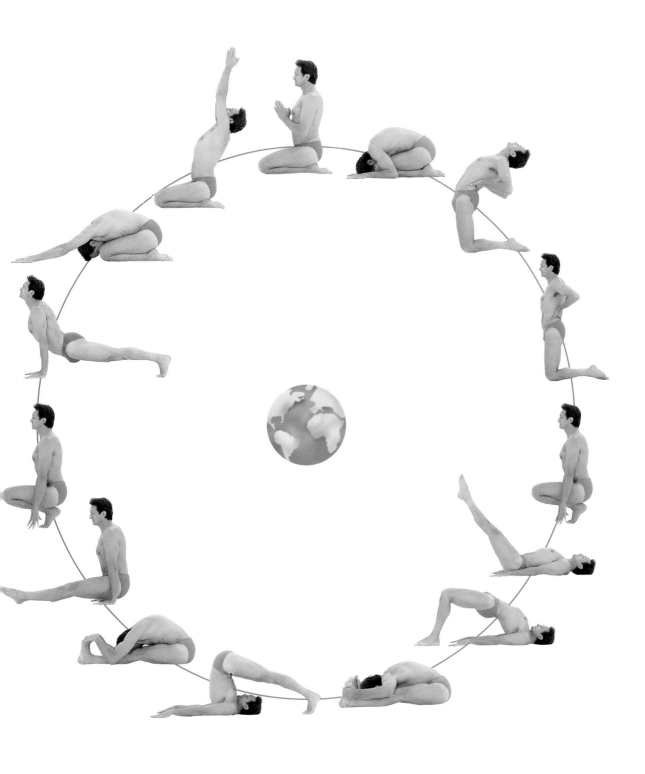

2. Sitting
Backward-Bending Pose

Inhale as you raise your arms over your head, *crossing your thumbs.* At the same time, drop your head back and bend backward from the hips bringing your arms back as far as you can. The arch extends from your lower back up to your fingertips. Look toward the ceiling. Exhale.

1. Prayer Pose

Inhale-exhale as you place your palms flat together and rest your underarms on your chest. Your forearms, wrists, and hands are kept in a straight line with thumbs crossed.

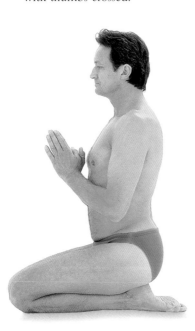

3. Half Tortoise Pose

Inhale-exhale as you bend forward, placing your palms on the ground. Your arms are parallel, elbows are locked, and your shoulders and spine are extended. Remain seated on your heels if you can. Rest your head on the ground, *elongating your spine and stretching your shoulders and arms.*

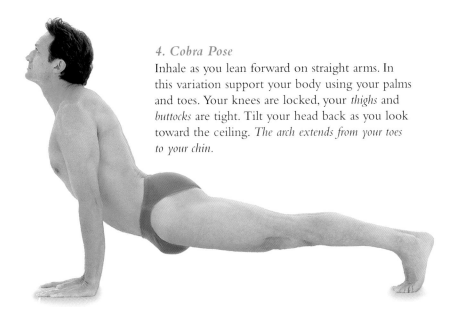

4. Cobra Pose

Inhale as you lean forward on straight arms. In this variation support your body using your palms and toes. Your knees are locked, your *thighs* and *buttocks* are tight. Tilt your head back as you look toward the ceiling. *The arch extends from your toes to your chin.*

5. Squatting Pose
Exhale as you lower your knees
to the floor and, with support
from your arms, sit back on
your toes.

6. Sitting Pose
Inhale-exhale as you sit down on
the floor, legs extended, arms at
your sides. As you sit, support your
body with your arms in order to
soften the landing.

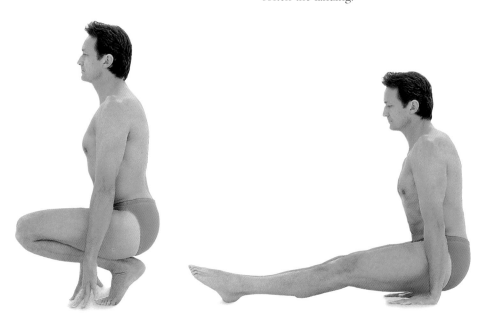

7. Sitting Hands-to-Feet Pose

Inhale as you raise your arms over your head
and exhale as you bend forward and grasp your
feet or lower legs, pulling your torso toward
your legs. *Lock your knees if you can.*

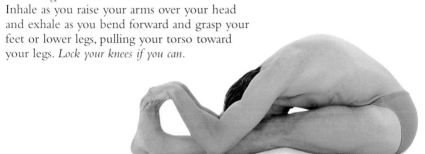

8. Plough Pose

Inhale-exhale as you release your grip while rolling back, legs
over your head. This is an uninterrupted motion. Support
your body with your straight arms kept flat on the floor.
Stretch your back. Keep your neck free of tension—only your
back should feel the stretch. Keep your legs together. (If you
have difficulty rolling back, support your body by placing
your palms on your hips.)

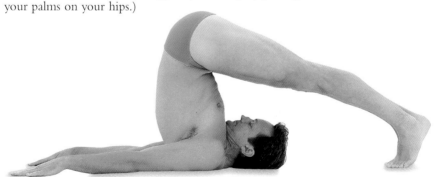

9. Sitting Legs–Apart Hands-to-Feet Pose
Inhale-exhale as you roll forward, legs spread wide. In an uninterrupted motion, bend forward and grasp your feet or lower legs from outside. *Pull your head and torso close to the floor by straightening your legs. Feel the stretch in your legs, back, and shoulders.*

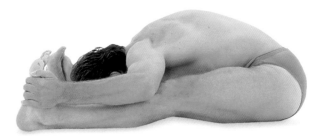

10. Bridge Pose
Inhale as you release your grip and lie back on the floor, arms straight and palms down. At the same time, bend your knees, bringing your heels toward your buttocks, and press your pelvis toward the ceiling. Your feet and knees are shoulder width apart, and your buttocks and back are tightened. *Feel the stretch in your thighs, pelvis, abdomen, and chest up to your neck.* (If you have difficulty with this pose, support your waist with your palms.)

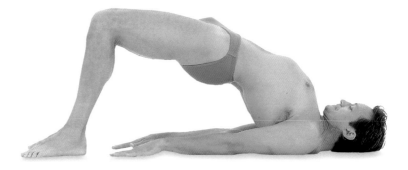

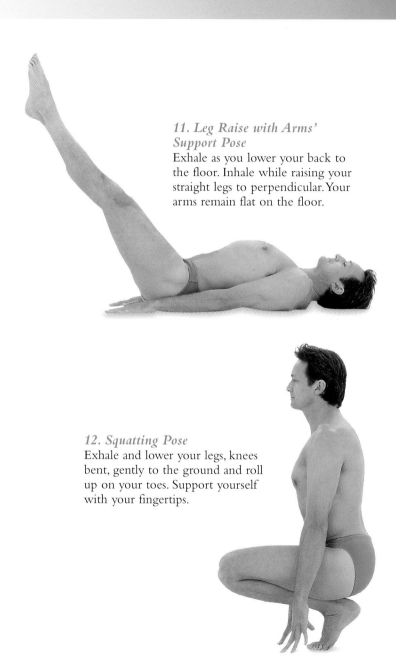

11. Leg Raise with Arms' Support Pose

Exhale as you lower your back to the floor. Inhale while raising your straight legs to perpendicular. Your arms remain flat on the floor.

12. Squatting Pose

Exhale and lower your legs, knees bent, gently to the ground and roll up on your toes. Support yourself with your fingertips.

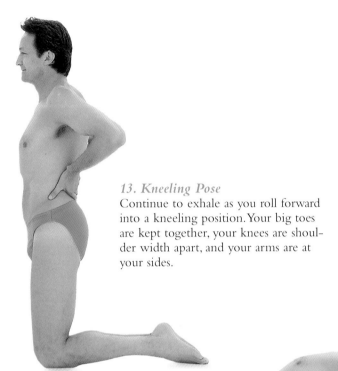

13. Kneeling Pose

Continue to exhale as you roll forward into a kneeling position. Your big toes are kept together, your knees are shoulder width apart, and your arms are at your sides.

14. Camel Pose

Inhale as you place your palms on your waist for support. Then bend backward, dropping your head. You will feel a strong stretch in your thighs, abdomen, chest, and throat. (If your neck is stiff or sensitive, do not drop your head back.)

Exhale as you raise your torso back to perpendicular. Sit down on your heels, placing your palms or fingertips on the floor at your sides and bringing your knees together.

15. Child Pose

Inhale-exhale as you lean forward on your thighs and rest with palms, lower arms, and head on the floor. (If you have difficulty resting on your thighs, spread your knees slightly.)

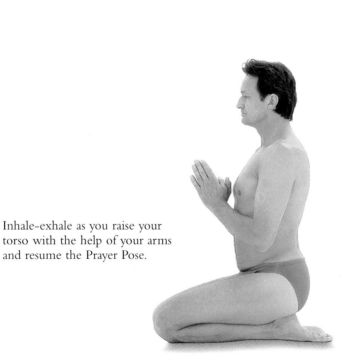

Inhale-exhale as you raise your torso with the help of your arms and resume the Prayer Pose.

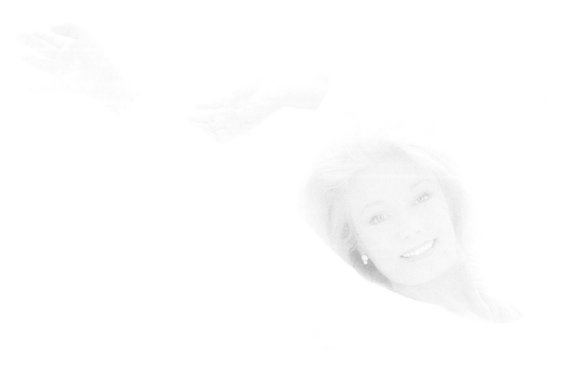

Salutation to the Sun

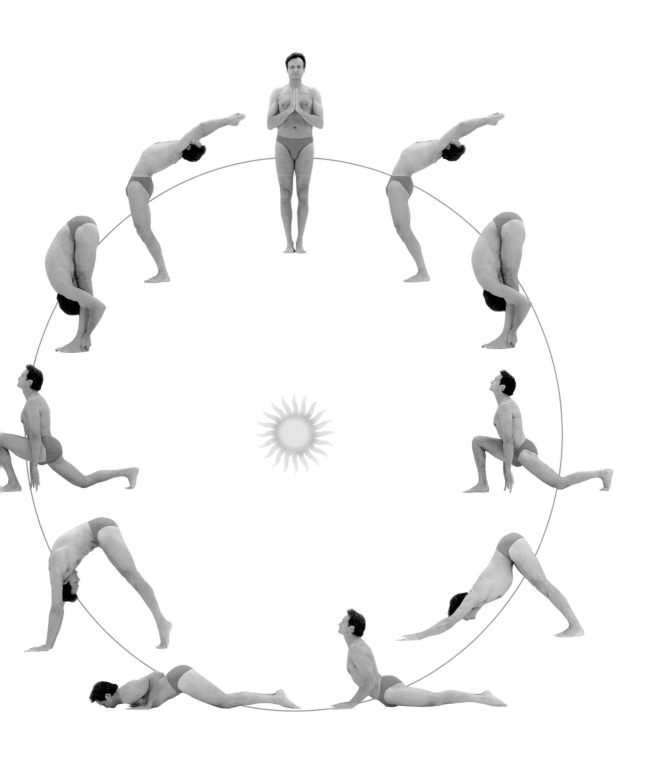

2. Standing
Backward–Bending Pose
Inhale as you raise your arms over your head, *crossing your thumbs.* At the same time, drop your head back and bend backward from your hips, legs straight, *knees locked, thighs and buttocks tightened.* The arch extends from the heels of your feet up to your fingertips. Look toward the ceiling. *Feel the stretch along the front of your body.*

1. Prayer Pose

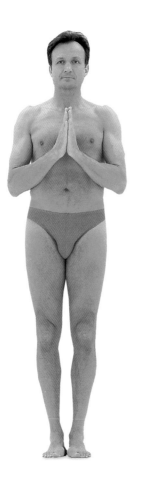

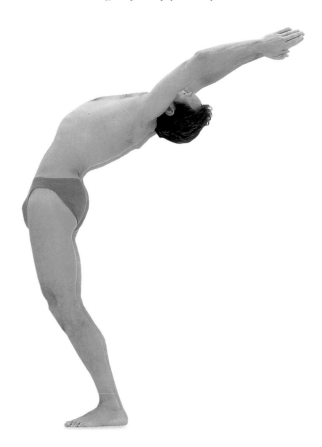

3. Standing
Hands-to-Feet Pose

Exhale as you return to perpendicular, arms and torso straight,
and continue to bend forward,
knees bent, grasping your heels
or lower legs and pulling your
head and body close to your legs,
gradually locking your knees. *Feel
the stretch in your calves, hamstrings,
buttocks, and back.*

4. Equestrian Pose on Right Leg

Inhale as you place your fingertips on the floor
on either side of your feet and take a big step
back with your right leg. Arch fully by pressing
your pelvis toward the floor, *straightening your right
leg*, tilting your head back, and directing your gaze
upward. *The arch extends from the toes of your right
foot up to your chin.* Exhale. (Your weight is on
your left foot and the toes of your right foot. Your
left foot should be flat on the floor. Do not lift
your heel. In the beginning you might keep your
right knee on the ground, but as you advance, lift
it by straightening that leg.)

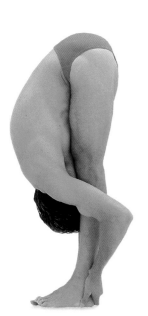

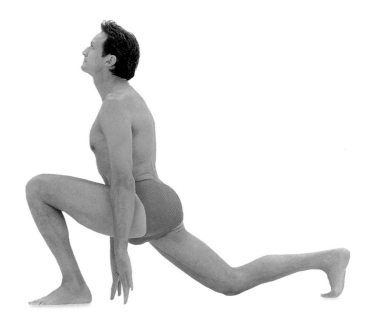

77

5. Cat Pose

Inhale as you place your palms on the floor, simultaneously stepping back with your left foot, placing it next to the right foot. At the same time, raise up on the balls of your feet, curl your back, and press your chin to your chest. Your elbows and knees are locked. *Feel the stretch from your toes to your shoulders.*

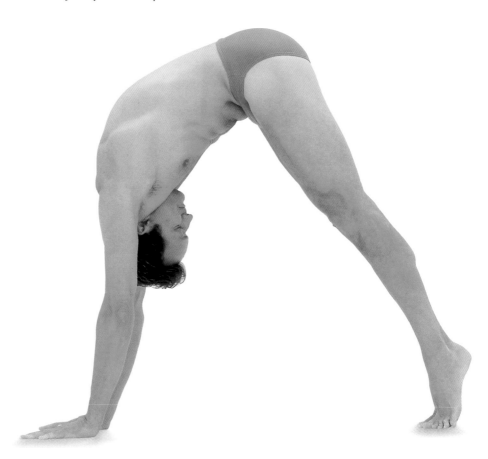

6. Salutation with Eight Limbs Pose

Exhale as you collapse gradually, in a controlled manner, to your knees, then onto the floor—but keep your pelvis off the floor. Only your toes, knees, palms, chest, and face should touch the ground.

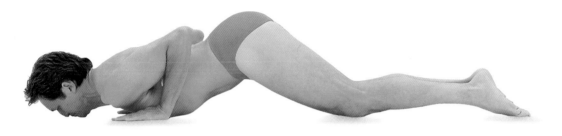

7. Cobra Pose

Inhale as you lock your knees and point your toes while raising your torso from your hips, supporting yourself with your arms, into a fully arched position. Your lower body remains flat on the floor, *your thighs and buttocks tightened. Feel the stretch from your toes to your chin.* Tilt your head back and direct your gaze toward the ceiling.

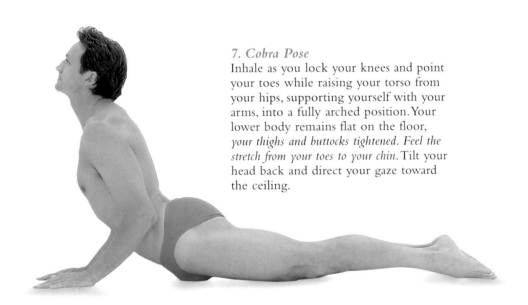

8. Downward Dog Pose

Exhale as you lift your body in a wavelike motion, supporting your weight on your hands and feet. Ultimately your knees and elbows will be locked, your back arched from the hips, and your head tilted back. Press your heels deliberately toward the floor. *Feel the stretch in the back of your legs, your buttocks, back, shoulders, and arms.*

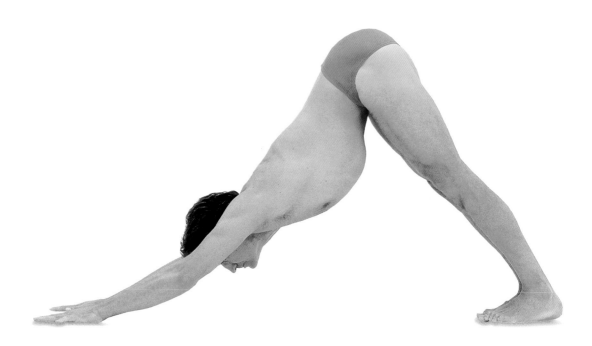

9. Equestrian Pose on Left Leg

Inhale as you raise up on your fingertips, stepping your right leg forward between your hands. Lower your pelvis toward the floor and resume the Equestrian Pose. *The arch extends from the toes of your left foot up to your chin.*

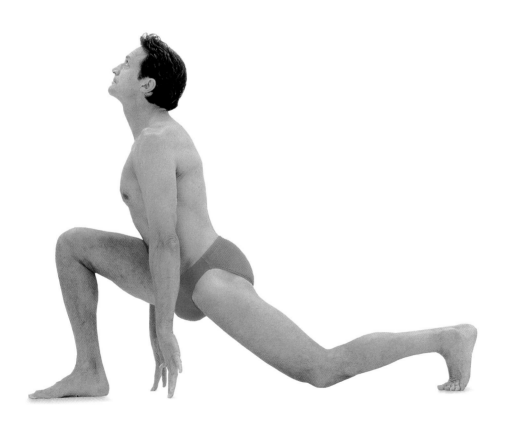

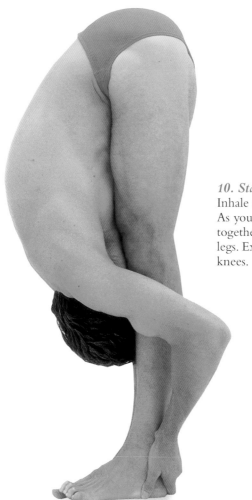

10. Standing Hands-to-Feet Pose
Inhale as you bring your left leg forward. As you crouch with knees bent and feet together, grasp your heels or your lower legs. Exhale as you gradually lock your knees.

11. Standing Backward-Bending Pose

Inhale as you raise your arms and torso to a perpendicular position, continuing into the Standing Backward-Bending Pose.

Exhale as you straighten your body and arms, resuming the Prayer Pose.

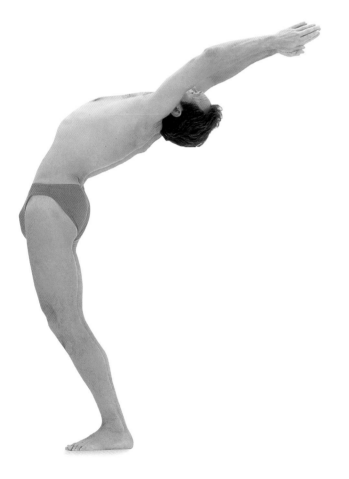

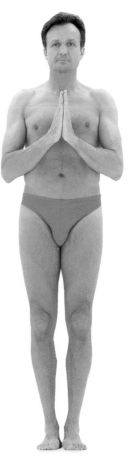

Salutation to the Moon

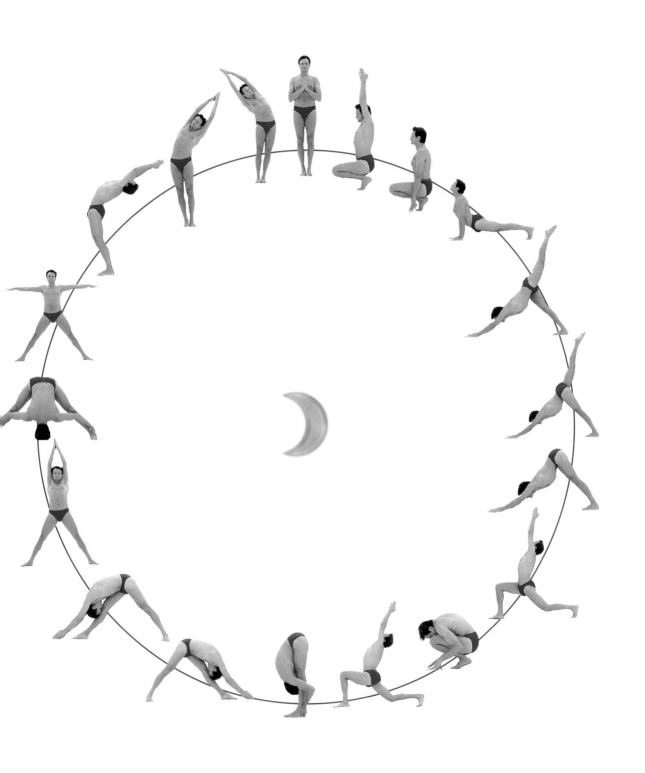

1. Prayer Pose

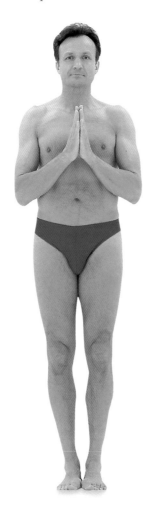

2. Half Moon Pose to the Right

Inhale as you lower your arms to your sides and raise them over your head in a lateral, circular motion. When your hands meet, press your palms together, thumbs crossed, arms straight, and reach toward the ceiling. Continue by bending to the right, moving your left hip to the left. Your knees are locked, and your thighs and buttocks are tightened. Your weight is distributed equally on both feet. Direct your gaze forward.

Exhale as you return to perpendicular.

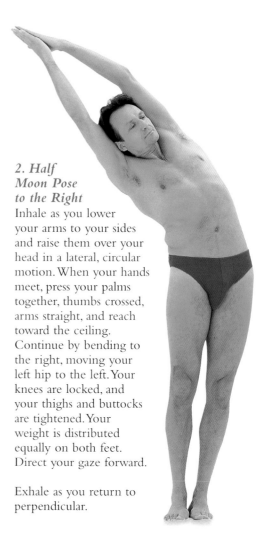

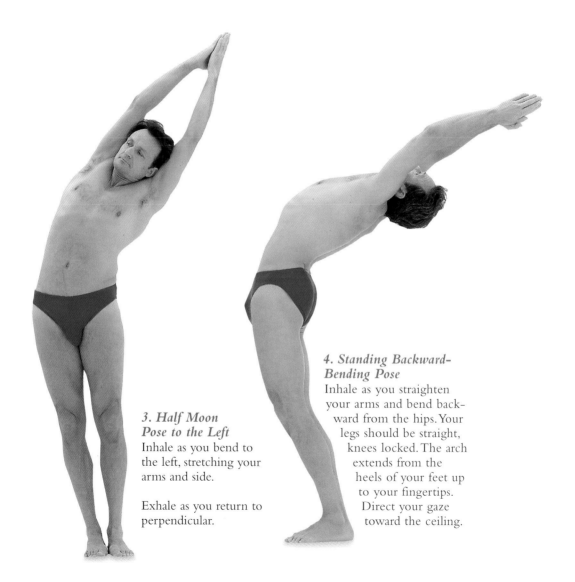

3. Half Moon
Pose to the Left
Inhale as you bend to the left, stretching your arms and side.

Exhale as you return to perpendicular.

4. Standing Backward-
Bending Pose
Inhale as you straighten your arms and bend backward from the hips. Your legs should be straight, knees locked. The arch extends from the heels of your feet up to your fingertips. Direct your gaze toward the ceiling.

5. Transition Pose 1
Exhale as you return to perpendicular. Inhale as you sidestep to the right, bringing straight arms down to shoulder level, parallel to the floor.

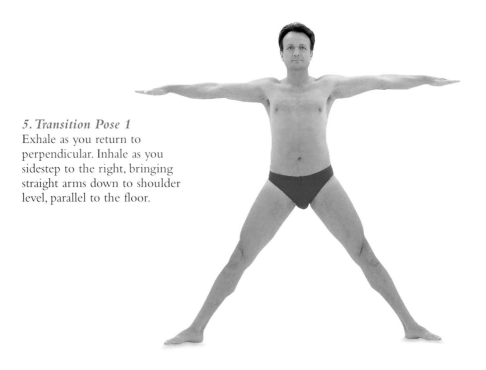

6. Standing Legs–Apart Hands-to-Feet Pose
Exhale as you bend forward, knees bent, and grasp your heels or lower legs, straightening your legs while pulling your torso between them. *Feel the stretch in your legs, torso, and shoulders.*

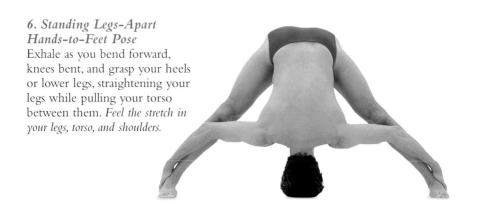

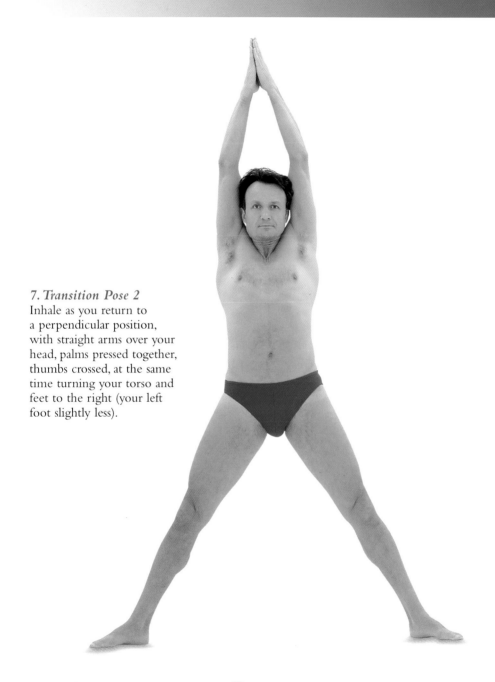

7. Transition Pose 2

Inhale as you return to a perpendicular position, with straight arms over your head, palms pressed together, thumbs crossed, at the same time turning your torso and feet to the right (your left foot slightly less).

8. Standing Head-to-Knee Pose to the Right

Exhale as you bend down, *left knee locked*, directing your forehead toward your right knee. At the same time, try to touch the floor with your fingertips as far ahead of your right foot as you can. *Gradually straighten your right leg, keeping your arms and fingers extended. Feel the stretch in your legs, back, shoulders, and arms.* (If this is too difficult, you might support yourself with your fingertips resting on the ground on either side of your right foot.)

Inhale-exhale as you return to perpendicular, turning your torso and feet straight ahead. Inhale as you turn to the left.

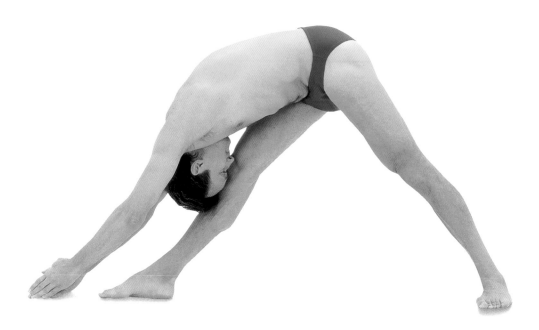

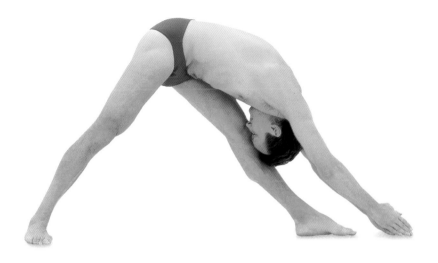

9. Standing Head-to-Knee
Pose to the Left
Exhale as you bend forward and down
to repeat this pose on the left.

Inhale as you return to perpendicular,
arms over your head, simultaneously
turning front and aligning your legs.

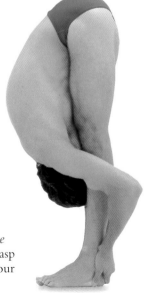

10. Standing Hands-to-Feet Pose
Exhale as you bend forward and grasp
your heels or lower legs and pull your
head and torso close to your legs.

11. Crescent Moon Pose on Right Leg

Inhale as you place your fingertips or palms on the floor beside your feet. At the same time take a big step back with your right, raising your torso and head—briefly assuming the Equestrian Pose. Still inhaling, bring your hands over your head, palms together, thumbs crossed. The arch extends from the toes of your right foot, through your leg and torso, and up to your fingertips. Your elbows are locked, your mouth is closed, your head is tilted back, and your gaze is directed upward. *Exhale.* (At first you might want to keep your knee on the floor. As you advance, lift it by straightening that leg.)

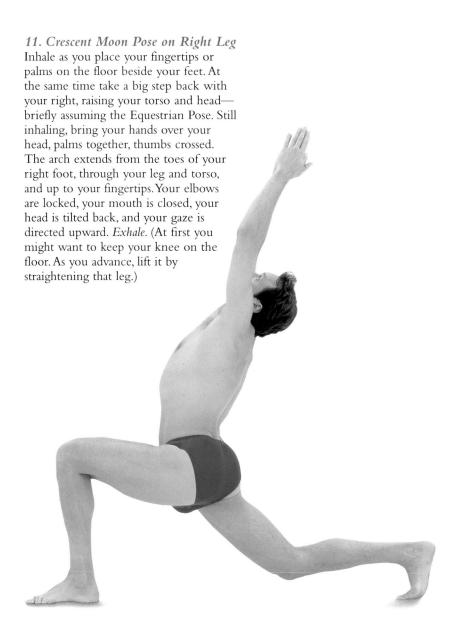

12. Squatting Pose
with Forward Bending

Inhale as you place your fingertips or palms on the floor and bring your right leg forward equal with your left. Your weight is supported by your toes and fingertips. *Your thighs are parallel to the floor.* Exhale as you bend forward, bringing your chest as close to your thighs as possible, fully stretching your back.

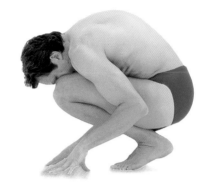

13. Crescent Moon Pose
on Left Leg

Inhale, raising your head and torso as you take a big step back with your left leg. Raise your arms over your head and stretch backward to resume the Crescent Moon Pose. Exhale.

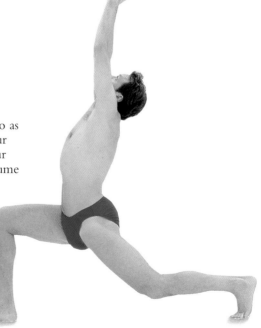

14. Downward Dog Pose
Inhale as you place your finger-tips back on the floor. Exhale as you step back with your right leg and arch your back from your hips. Remember to keep your heels on the floor.

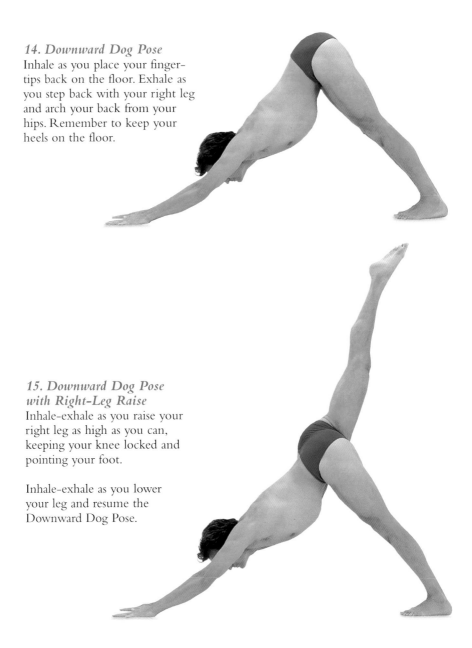

15. Downward Dog Pose with Right-Leg Raise
Inhale-exhale as you raise your right leg as high as you can, keeping your knee locked and pointing your foot.

Inhale-exhale as you lower your leg and resume the Downward Dog Pose.

16. Downward Dog Pose with Left-Leg Raise

Inhale-exhale as you raise your left leg as high as you can, keeping your knee locked and pointing your foot.

Inhale-exhale as you lower your leg and resume the Downward Dog Pose.

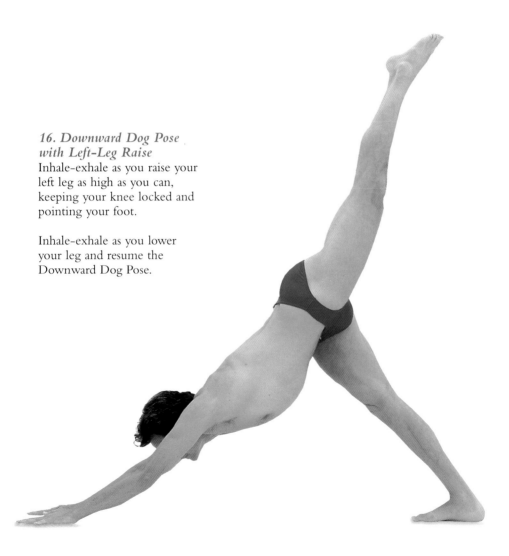

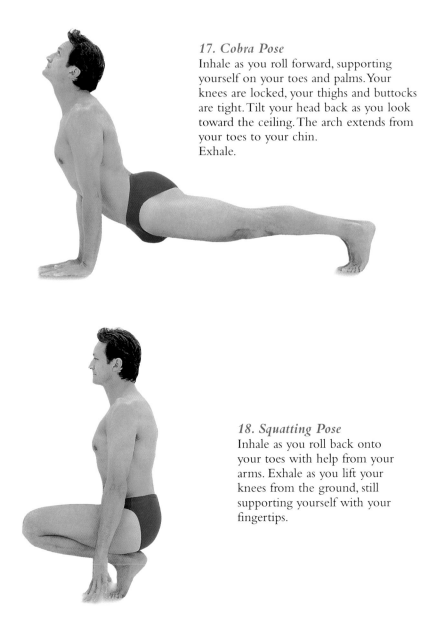

17. Cobra Pose
Inhale as you roll forward, supporting yourself on your toes and palms. Your knees are locked, your thighs and buttocks are tight. Tilt your head back as you look toward the ceiling. The arch extends from your toes to your chin.
Exhale.

18. Squatting Pose
Inhale as you roll back onto your toes with help from your arms. Exhale as you lift your knees from the ground, still supporting yourself with your fingertips.

19. Squatting Pose
with Arms over the Head

Inhale-exhale as you raise your arms over your head, palms together, thumbs crossed. Your elbows should be locked, your back straight, *and your thighs parallel to the floor. Feel the stretch in your torso, shoulders, and arms*. (If you have difficulty balancing on your toes, resume the Squatting Pose with your fingertips on the floor.)

Inhale as you stand up, simultaneously bringing your hands to your chest and resuming the Prayer Pose. Exhale. Take two steps forward, *right leg first*, to resume the starting position.

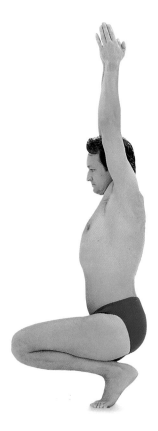

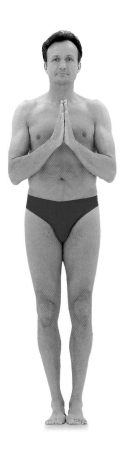

Sitting-Relaxing Deep Breathing

---

*T*his cooling-down exercise will slow the heartbeat and promote relaxation.

Sit down on your heels, as in the Prayer Pose, but with your palms resting on your thighs. Your back is straight, and your gaze is directed forward. Inhale deeply but easily through your nose and exhale evenly through your mouth. During inhalation your abdomen should expand; during exhalation, it should contract.

Inhale. Exhale.
Inhale through the nose.
Exhale through the mouth.
Inhale. Exhale.

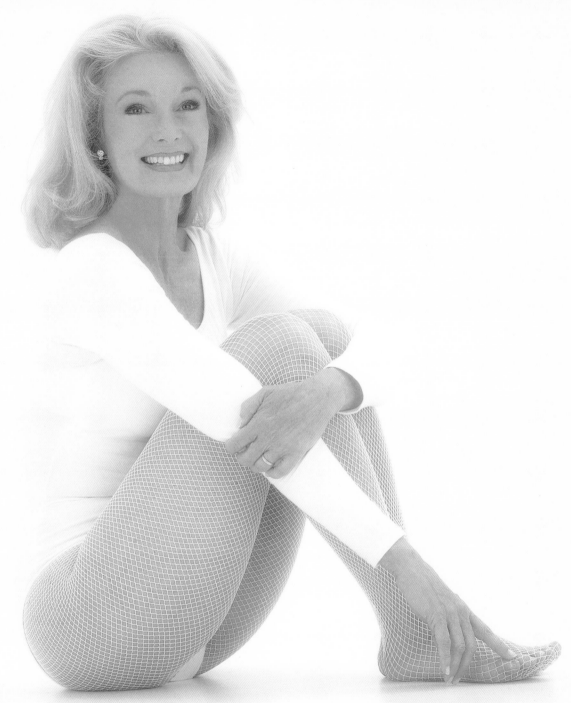

Inhale. Exhale.

Now lie on your back in Corpse Pose, breathing quietly through your nose. Your arms should rest comfortably at your sides, palms up. Your heels should be eight to ten inches apart. Allow your feet to fall to the sides. Keep your head in line with your torso, bringing your chin slightly down and directing your gaze slightly forward. As you continue to breathe quietly and evenly, place your right palm on your abdomen, your thumb over your navel, and monitor the rise and fall of your abdomen. Inhale and exhale four to six times. During inhalation, your abdomen should rise. During exhalation it should fall.

Inhale. Exhale.
Inhale through the nose.
Exhale through the nose.
Inhale. Exhale.
Inhale. Exhale.

Resume the Corpse Pose by placing your right hand on the floor. Allow calmness and serenity to pervade your body as you rest in this position.

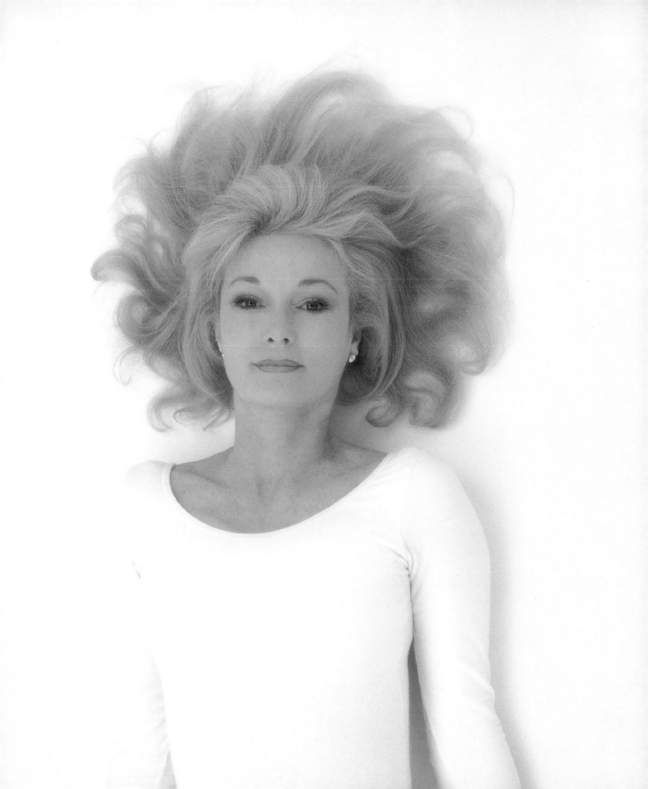

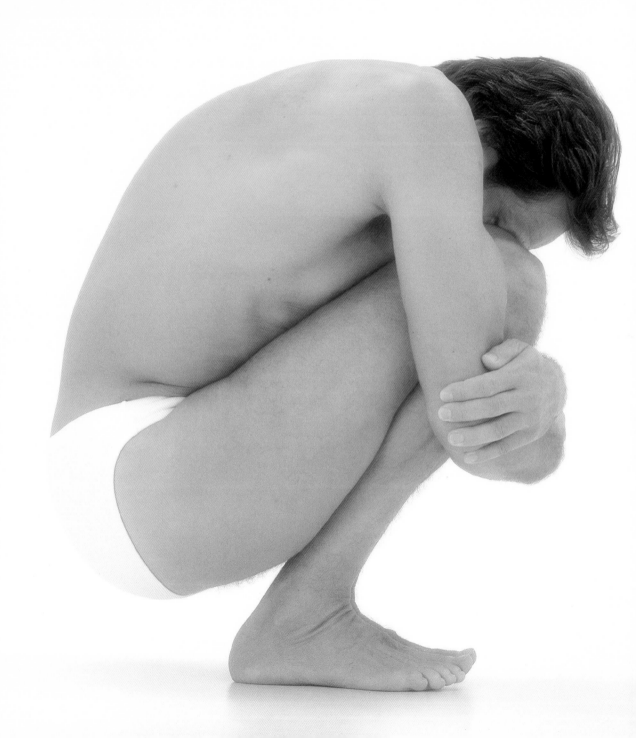

For a basic program do each cycle twice before going on to the next one. For a really strong aerobic workout, repeat each cycle three or four times. If your goal is stretching and strengthening only, go slowly and prolong the poses. This will allow you to learn the poses accurately. It is important to be precise. During slow cycles, always breathe continuously and evenly. Just be sure when to exhale and inhale at the beginning and end of the poses. After you memorize the poses and cycles, you can become your own instructor. You will decide the intensity and duration of your workout.